Simplify Your Health **Hydrate**

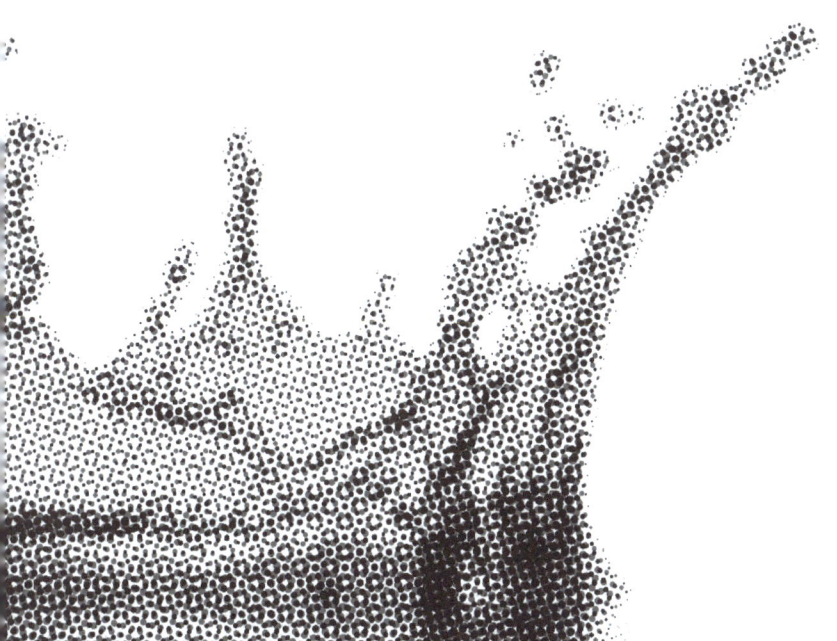

foreword

Living on the edge between different opinions, we examine the world of water marketing and scientific research.

Some will agree and some will disagree with opinions presented in this book, which will add fuel for discussing the possibilities, bringing us closer to a better understanding.

Simplify Your Health Hydrate

Written by Timothy Nicely
Copy Editor - Stefanie "Schui" Schumacher
Science Editor - Michael Rabinowitz, PhD
Chemistry Editor - Niles Smith
Cover Photo courtesy of Nao Magami
Designed in Los Angeles, California
Simplify Your Health Publishing
© 2011, 2013 Nicely. All Rights Reserved.
Distributed by OverUnity Creative, LLC

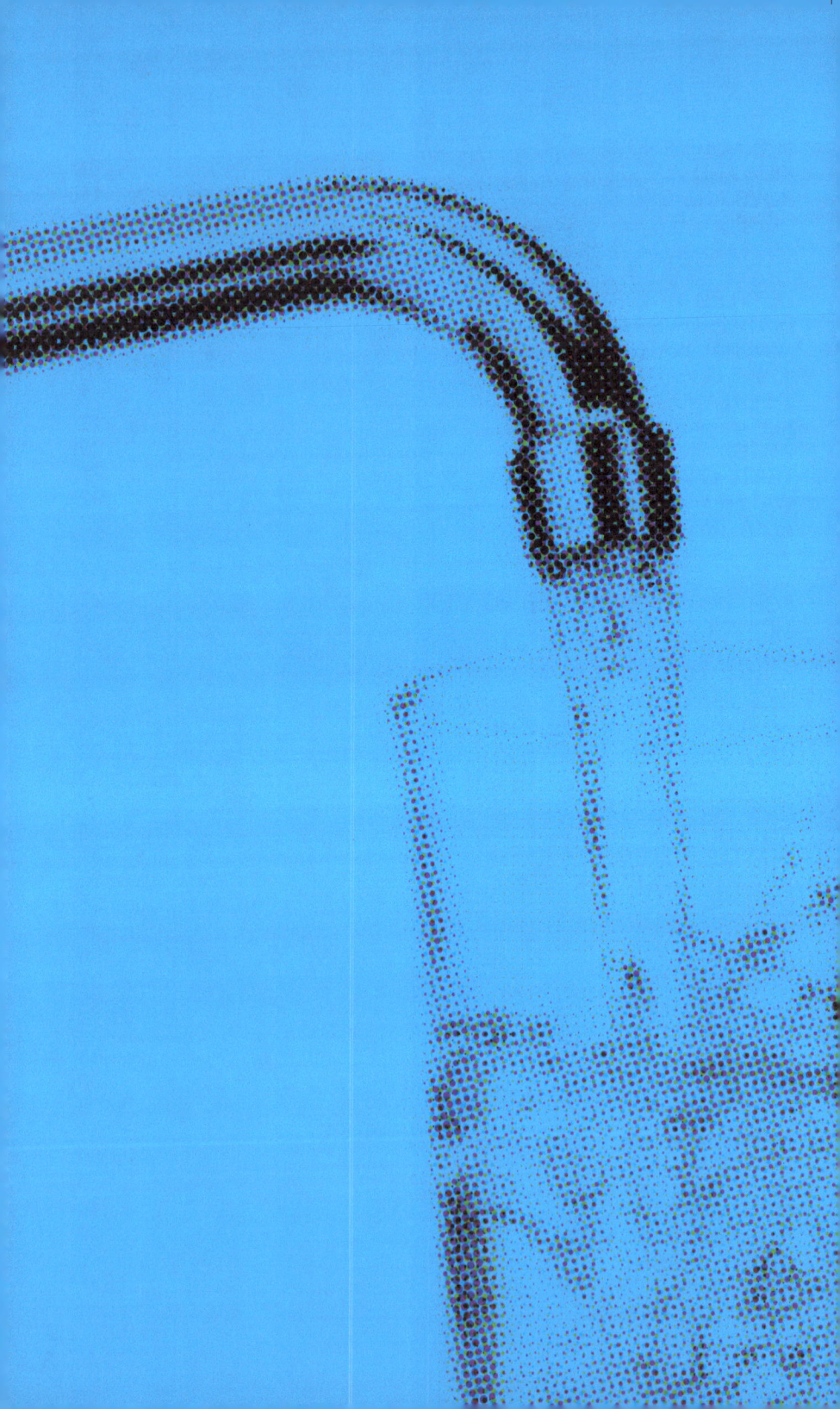

introduction

A person does not have to completely change their lifestyle to improve the quality of it.

This book does not aspire to change your way of life. It only strives to give the reader more clarity over the confusion powered by deceptive marketing or misinformation presented on the Internet or in other media.

We are not opposed to medical technologies; instead we applaud the advancement of science while focusing on current embellishments of personal or professional opinions and various fragmented researched statistics regarding water.

The author's primary interest in health was influenced when science proved that our bodies are designed to heal themselves. Scientific research further verifies exactly which crucial elements are needed to make healing possible.

Ultimately, a full spectrum of most elements are what our Immune System requires to enable our body to heal. Yet even though there are numerous professionals who evaluate research studies, there is always a controversy between those who agree and those who do not.

We will explore those conflicting opinions over documented research statistics and possible reasons for perplexing differences amongst seasoned physicians and other professionals.

The author feels that health and science is a perfect marriage to scrutinize health controversies, especially since science has already confirmed the link between diseases and the missing elements that allow them to exist.

This simplified approach to health is meant to encourage us to be more aware of what to believe and how it applies to our own health. Draw your own conclusions. Welcome to Simplify Your Health.

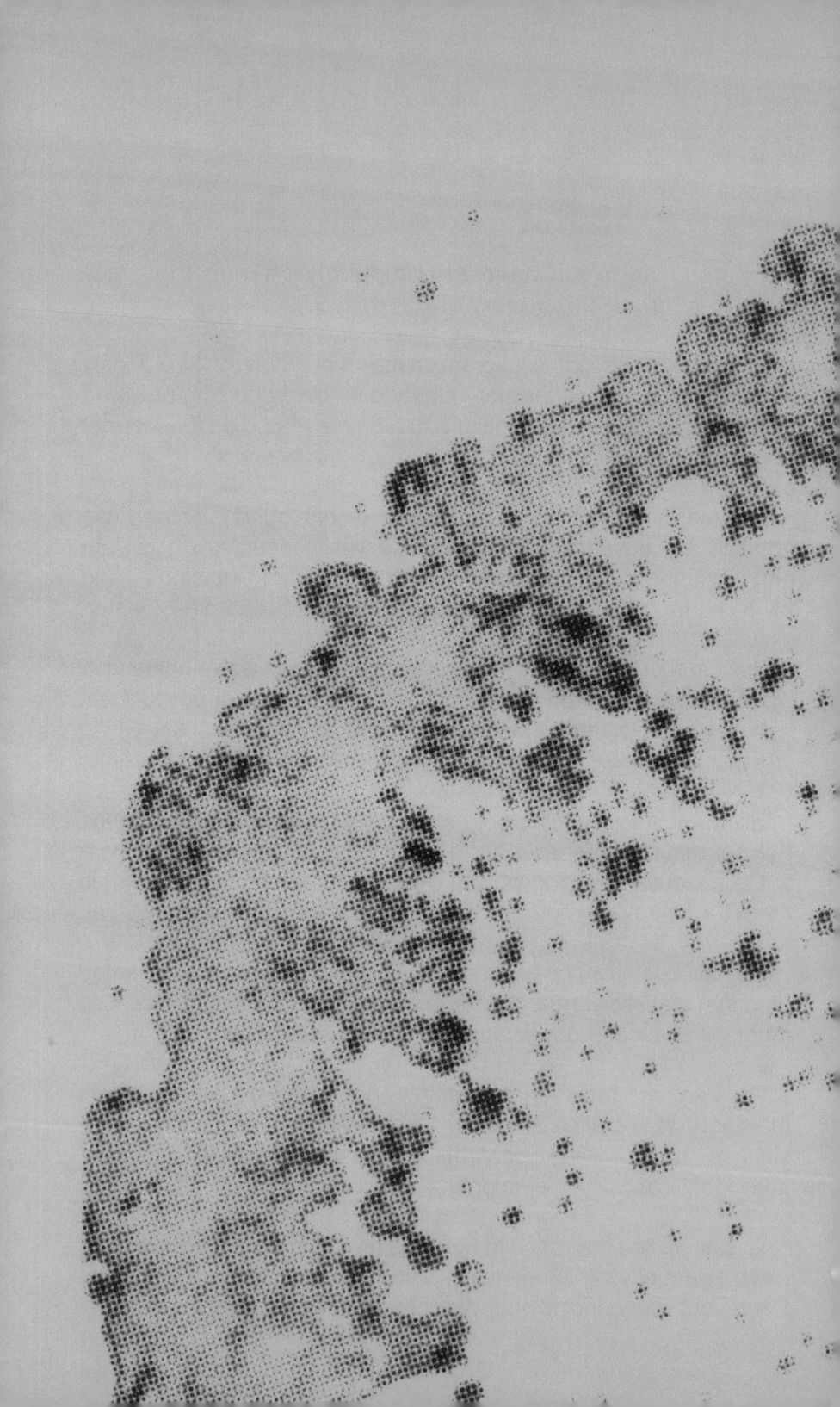

hydrate

For the last three decades we have been overloaded with health data. To simplify, I began to focus on elements that are absolutely essential for a healthy life such as water, real salt, minerals and phyto-chemicals.These basic elements have been missing from our diet in general, either by accident or by design.

The bottom line defense against disease is a strong functional immune system. Whether you choose doctors or alternative medicine, it will be your immune system that heals you, but it needs water to function.

While growing up we have been told to drink eight glasses of water a day, but usually without knowing why we should do this. Hydrate unravels and clarifies the reasons why and examines conflicting research on water.

Water is a basic delivery system for nutrition, electrical impulses and body mechanisms. The more our cells get hydrated, the less chance our bodies will become diseased.

A telling sign of proper water hydration and cell functioning is evident in the health, glow and vibrancy of one's skin, which receives one-third of all blood from the heart. The skin is our largest organ and is responsible for a fourth of our body's detoxification by eliminating up to two pounds of waste per day in the form of sweat, oils and shedding of the outer layer of dead skin. Having dehydrated dry skin is not a healthy state.

Water is the elixir of life, and now the most recent data reveals that water may also be a living organism with a consciousness that responds to our attitudes. This sounds strange but may now be provable.

The present scientific definition of an "organism" is any living system of animals, plants, fungus or microorganisms, plus any molecules that show signs of life. After decades of worldwide water research, this vital element may now qualify as an organism. (Institute of Science in Society - http://www.i-sis.org.uk/WaterRemembers.php)

Can water routinely do what it does in our bodies without it being a living organism? We will explore that question.

I first became aware of the importance of water back in 1973, when I began drinking bottled water. Yet, I did not realize how important water really was until years later when I awoke one morning with severe pain in my knee. I had never experienced anything that painful in my leg before. The pain continued for weeks while I tried various remedies.

It was during that ordeal when I came across a book "Your Body's Many Cries For Water" by Doctor Batmanghelidj, who had discovered water therapy when incarcerated in an Iranian jail waiting to be executed. When it was his turn to be judged, he presented his notes and was granted a delay to continue his research. He was released and escaped from Iran. The world is more enriched by his innovative thinking, as his courageous journey brought him to America and taught him how to better relieve the suffering of thousands.

I discovered that although I had been drinking a quart of carbonated water daily for years, apparently it was not enough. The quenching bubbles had given me a false sense of hydration. I was only consuming half of what my body weight needed to function properly, and so dehydration finally caught up with me.

The doctor had used water successfully to improve health in clients for more than 25 years. He proved through clinical tests and patient histories that "you may not be sick, just thirsty." That thought made so much sense it drew me further into the world of water. He felt that to treat dehydration with medications is not the answer, pointing out that Chronic Cellular Dehydration leads to pain and death. Plus, if we have an unknown disease, our bodies may likely be severely dehydrated.

Carole Punt's "Electricity For Health" points out that there are 100 trillion cells that are separated by a watery fluid. This fact also paints a clear picture of the importance of drinking enough water for a healthy functioning body.

After following Dr. Batmanghelidj's water paradigm, eliminating my knee pain in three days, I decided to interview him for a magazine book review. He consented and in appreciation I sent him a packet of Celtic Sea Salt, now available on his website. The importance of this particlular salt will surprise many who believe sodium is real salt ("Sea Salt's Hidden Powers" by Dr. Jacques de Langre).

By using his new water paradigm, my life changed. Continuing my daily water consumption and learning as much about this man's work was a final link needed to simplify my health.

Now, nearly two decades later, I still have not experience any recurrence of knee pain.

When our bodies experience pain, it may just be a water shortage. Prescription drugs can cover up dehydration signals. This is not always good as physical pain alerts us that there is something wrong.

Take notice of the people who walk around with pain in their legs or in other parts of their body. More often than not they will have chapped lips, a sign of chronic dehydration.

the nose knows

When I first needed to increase my water consumption, I had to reaccustom my taste buds to the liquid. Within a few days, I began liking water again and noticed that there is a subtle taste to good water. There was no problem in drinking two to three quarts a day, until my lips regained their moisture and the knee pain was gone.

Why do we tend not to drink water as much as tasty juices

or sodas? It is our nose that first determines how much we eat or drink. When we drink juices or sugar water, our nose tells our body it is food, so we continue to drink more until we are full. When we consume water, our nose detects "non-food" so we then tend to quench only our immediate thirst.

If you must fool your nose to consume more water, try adding an unsqueezed slice of lemon to the glass of water so your nose can detect the citrus aroma while drinking.

kids & water

For several years I volunteered in an after-school program with kids. Many of these children were chronically dehydrated. Some had severely cracked lips. This disturbed me. I explained when-ever I could that this may lead to "Dis-Ease" later on in life.

In every schoolyard I had visited, there were soda machines. Al-though now, some schools with concerned administrators and parents have removed those machines.

Children are destroying their bodies by drinking too much soda and not enough water. I would tell them "drink water!" The kids would often reply, "I drink soda and juice all the time!" Soda and juice are not the same as water! But that bubbly sugar fix from a frosty soda container on a hot day is too much of a lure for most of us.

It seems that this early addictive behavior pattern begins when we are babies and are given our first taste of sugar. Refined sugar makes you feel better, until you crash and need another quick sugar fix. Strong hooks are then planted deep within our cell memory and become part of who we are. We are a society of soda drinkers rather than water drinkers.

I grew up a dedicated sugar addict. By the time I was a teenager, I had very little strength in my muscles. It magnified my lazy reputation. What I did not know then is that insulin deficiency and insulin resistance are both a blood sugar problem (www.endocrineweb. com/diabetes). After the initial rush of a sudden burst of sugar, my muscles always felt weak. Back then this feeling was called "lazy bones".

When we consume too much soda instead of drinking water, it may affect the cerebrospinal fluid (CSF) within the skull and spine. This clear, colorless fluid surrounds the brain to cushion it. It is made of water ("The Brain and Nervous System" http://health.how-stuffworks.com/brain-nervous-system-ga1.htm).

Adequate water in and around our brain protects us while facilitating concentration. Students need water to focus better. Educating a young malfunctioning dry brain does not work favorably for the youth struggling to think clearly.

boys & girls

When I speak with some women about dehydration some of them respond, "it's easier for guys to drink lots of water because they can go to the bathroom almost anywhere. Women can't." While there is a certain truth in that logic, I ask those women to consider what is more inconvenient, a medical condition or finding a place to relieve ourselves?

hereditary

Dr. Batmanghelidj told me that dehydration problems could be passed on to your offspring. This made sense to me as many people have told me that their present medical condition runs in their family. I suggest it is passed-on deficiencies, which gets worse with every generation. Unhealthy habits increase our hereditary deficient biological destiny.

That, combined with learned behaviors of not drinking enough water, can devastate a body before it is fully-grown. Research absolutely shows that dehydration and disease go hand-in-hand, which may be also a part of a person's predisposition to heredity illness.

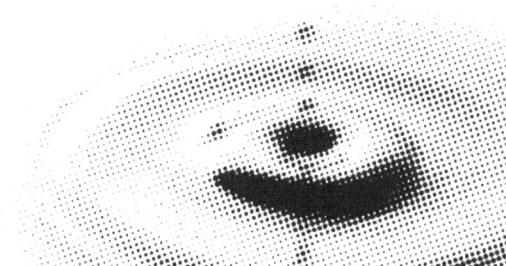

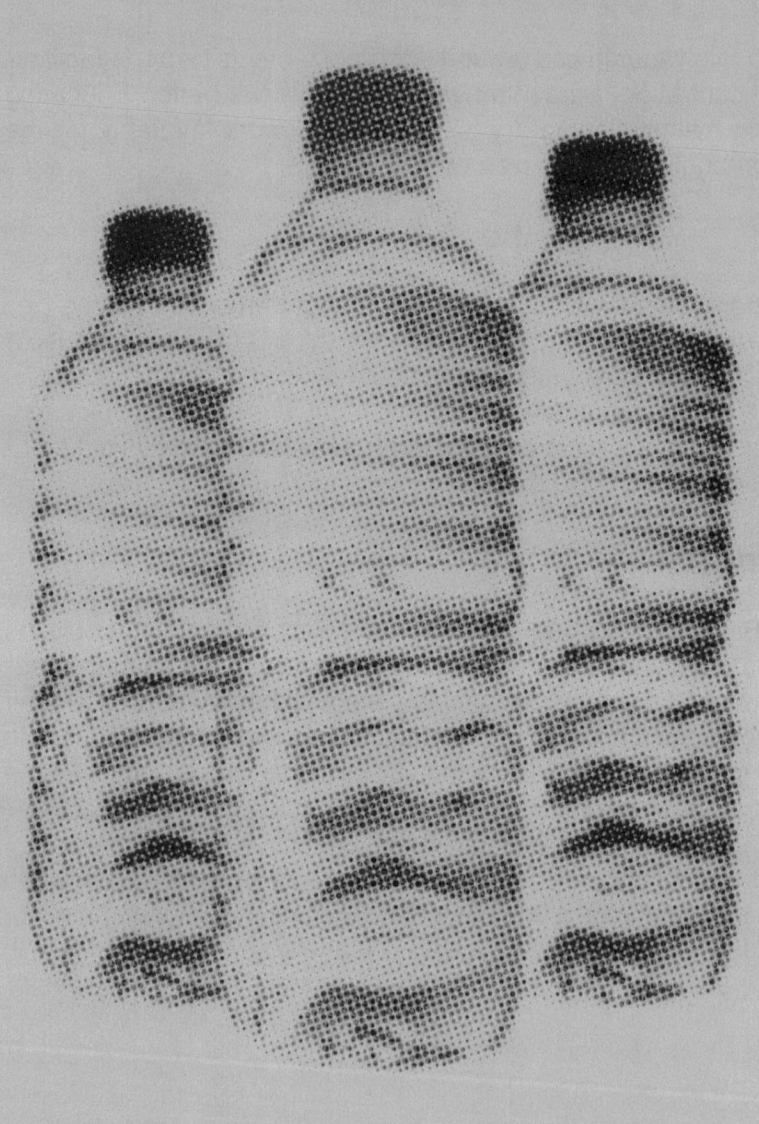

water supply

bottled water

A billion dollar industry, bottled water verbiage may be partly true in some cases but a lot of it is printed with a vague and seemingly useful arrangement of words designed to fool us. It's called deceptive marketing.

To be more certain that the bottled water is not just from an inadequately filtered tap water system, first read the label. Notice the water processing information. If it is not there, be apprehensive. A number of popular water companies are using municipal tap water, yet are allowed to claim it to be natural, spring, glacial, pure, premium, etc.

Much of the bottled water available has now been proven not to be as healthy as once assumed. Apart from the water itself, the plastic container is considered dangerous and a source of contaminants. The safest plastic container has a #1 inside a triangle shape on the bottom.

We hear warnings to keep some plastics out of microwave ovens or even the sun. Media reports also have cautioned us against freezing water in a plastic bottle. Cooked or frozen, contaminates may leach out of the plastic into the water.

The National Research Center for Women and Families states that the FDA should not be telling us plastic food containers are safe until proven so. The National Toxicology Program lists numerous bisphenol A (BPA) studies that show it to be a hazardous contaminate which can alter human development. The American Chemistry Council (ACC) says BPA is safe, yet the FDA's science advisors point out that over 100 published studies proving the danger of this substance is being ignored by decision makers. The FDA has only recently expressed concern over the safety of this hormone-like chemical ("Reversing itself, FDA expresses concerns over health risks from BPA" Washington Post - 01/16/2010).

The Environmental Working Group (EWG) also cites 293 studies finding harmful effects from BPA. As well, the Center for Disease Control and Prevention has found this chemical in 95% of Americans tested.

A bit of good news concerning plastic that was discovered by a high school student from Canada. This young mind has identified the two strains of bacteria that make plastic decompose. This innovative thinker believes that the two newly discovered microbes found in nature, can accelerate plastic deterioration from 1000 years down to three months. Proving again, possibilities for solutions are unlimited.

I use a stainless steel container to carry my water in.

distilled vs. filtering systems

Distilled water is definitely purified, but for years I have heard that distilled water flushes out nutrients from the body. The reality is that distilled water helps to absorb nutrients already in the body. When inorganic minerals are flushed, the water's ability to absorb whatever is left in your cells increases ("Fit for Life" by Harvey & Marilyn Diamond). Apparently, the good stuff does not easily leach out.

Distilled and de-ionized are the most common forms of purified water. Reverse Osmosis is also a purifying method that works by using pressure to force water through a membrane, leaving impurities behind. The Reverse Osmosis process may also utilize ozonation from ultraviolet lights that have been proven to kill certain pathogens.

Various filters can remove Fluoride, Arsenic, Lead, Chlorine, Heavy Metal, Bacteria, Zeomic, Noxious Odor, Calcium, Trihalomethanes, Suspended Solids, Cryptosporidium, Parasite (Cysts), Waterborne Fly Virus, Organic Compounds, E-Coli, Sulfates, and Sediment.

14

Distilling purifies water which has many clinical and industrial uses, yet drinking distilled water may not be the healthiest way to hydrate since it also creates an acid base through the purifying process. (See "pH Balance" section.)

mineral water

Are minerals in water really that useful except to change acid water to alkaline? Can we assimilate minerals other than by eating plants? Plants absorb inorganic minerals from good soil, but many plants do not absorb enough to supply our bodies with essential nutrients ("Nutrient Changes in Vegetables and Fruits, 1951 to 1999" - http://www.ctv.ca/servlet/articlenews/story/CTVNews/20020705/favaro_nutrients_chart_020705). Yet it seems this is the only way to receive absorbable minerals in a natural way.

There is a company selling mineral water from petrified plant sources located in a prehistoric valley. This "special" water is extracted from humus scale reportedly full of prehistoric mineral-rich plant nutrients. This same substance can be purchased inexpensively from any hydroponics store and it is not prehistoric.

This company originally claimed that there are no less than 60 plant-derived colloidal minerals from their humus scale. A full mineral spectrum should be higher. I once met the author of this humus concoction at a convention. When I mentioned real Celtic Salt with a full spectrum of minerals, he defensively interrupted with "Our product has more minerals!" Maybe by now he has done the math.

So, although humus percolation using plant debris may create absorbable minerals, do these minerals last millions of years in humus scale form? Some may in small amounts, but the majority of minerals in this product are from their own mineral blend. Taking that added blend into account can only mean that very few of their minerals come from prehistoric sources. **Read those labels.**

How can minerals in an inorganic state end up organic in water without going through a plant? According to RawFoodExplained. com, they cannot. Live plants are the only natural way to convert inorganic minerals to organic, which then makes them absorbable. Organic minerals come from food.

Tap water generally has inorganic minerals in it that are not absorbable. Their presence can cause some diseases from the poisoning of the intestines ("What experts say about distilled water" AquaTechnology.net). Drinking too much tap water with inorganic minerals may be a hazard to your health.

ionized water

Electron Energized Technology is spreading fast. Known as Ionized Water, the machines create high alkaline liquid by separating the acid from the alkaline ions. One ionized water company makes available a combo filter of Calcium Carbonate and Coral Calcium for their system, which increases the alkaline level. Another manufacturer with a very overpriced machine even injects Calcium Carbonate directly into the water to increase the pH reading.

Although the chemical Calcium Carbonate is listed as toxic by the Pesticide Action Network North America, authentic food grade Coral Calcium is healthy. The Periodic Table of the Elements lists Calcium as Ca, while MedLinePlus from the National Library of Medicine, lists Calcium Carbonate as $CaCO_3$ and warns consumers that if they overdose on it, to call a Poison Center. Some anti-coral calcium websites claim these two elements are the same.

Most ocean corals have small Polyps living in them. The Polyps produce a hard skeleton of calcium carbonate around its base. These Coral Polyps are small marine invertebrate animals that eat zooplankton (marine larvae). Then the Crown-of-Thornes Starfish, Parrot Fish and other animals eat the corals. ("Coral Reefs in the South Pacific Handbook" by Dr. Michael King). A Data Analysis Sheet for the food grade coral calcium I use, lists 69 trace minerals in the coral pre-digested by the fish. This seems to account for the difference between the two elements since calcium carbonate does not have all these minerals in it.

After researching acid/alkaline data, it became obvious that diseases live well in an acidic environment. According to BioNatural. com.au and other research sites, degenerative problems are associated with excess acid in the body. So, is alkaline water better for us?

One of the reasons why an alkaline system is vital for a healthy body is that alkaline tissue reportedly holds more oxygen than acidic tissues. This is important since oxygen keeps us alive and well. There are numerous supporting facts in favor of alkaline, yet this subject continues to remain loaded with confusing and conflicting opinions.

In conclusion, ionized machines do separate acid from alkaline but they are also dependent on a filtering system to clean up some of the toxins.

So, no matter what an alkaline Water Ionizer Technology Manufacture states about the superiority of their machine, and although the machines produce water with high alkaline levels, they do not reduce much of the toxins in the tap water being processed by the machines. Plus, it is important to remember the "slightly" alkaline rule -- With these machines you may over-do the alkaline needed, which is medically known to potentially lead to other imbalances and complications.

According to an industry source at a busy water store that sells ionized water (and their highly over-priced, out-dated technology which is being dumped on America using multi-level marketing), the ionization process only lasts for several weeks. It takes longer than that to get bottled water distributed into the market place.

During water shelf life testing I found there are different life spans for a wide variety of alkaline waters. After a few months several popular brands of alkaline water changed back to an acidic state. This can be proven at home by conducting your own pH tests by measuring water samples over several weeks or months.

pH balance

To test for the pH of water, pool stores should have liquid drops for basic color indications of water pH, while health stores usually carry measurement strips for body fluid readings.

A neutral body reading is pH 7. Normal is near 7.4 pH, which is considered slightly alkaline. Below 7 begins a slide into an acidic state.

There is a popular but expensive water on the market that claims it is electrically modified which reduces the size of the micro-clusters, which allegedly gives water the ability to penetrate deeper into our cells and provide more hydration. This is a popular brand of water but, again, this "purified water" is acidic when tested, which they claim is better for us.

Scientific reports show that alkaline water absorbs into the body better than acidic water, so their "acid" claims are hard to believe. Also, although micro-clusters are allegedly the key to better absorption, both sides of this issue claim the same clustering results. More confusion.

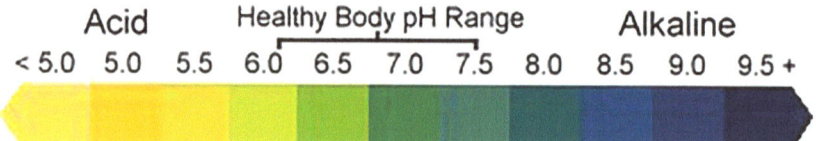

So if low pH (acid) water is as good as their promotion, then why do our bodies hold onto such heavy metals as mercury, lead and cadmium when it is in an acidic state? As well, bacteria and viruses are known to thrive better in an over-acidic body.

Though acidic water kills germs in the outer world, the acid pH of our bodies is more complex. Our bodies are designed for alkaline but acid is needed for proper function (TheWolfeClinic.com "The Importance of Your Body's pH Balance"). This presents two different body needs, which make the conflicting research scenario more comprehensible.

So, a slightly alkaline system is what our cells and tissues need for health, but our digestive system and urinary tract should be slightly acidic. The key word here for both is "slightly", which creates a balanced pH level.

For proper function on a cellular level, the cell interior is alkaline. This is where the power production of our bodies function best in a pool of alkaline water. A cell's exterior fluid is saline, alkaline and minerals.

When we drink alkaline water, it raises the stomach pH, which activates the production of Hydrochloric Acid for digestion while releasing bicarbonate into the bloodstream. The necessity of bicarbonate on health is well documented as the loss of bicarbonate may contribute to the accumulation of excess acid, which then contributes to cholesterol problems, fatty acids, uric acid and kidney stones.

On the other hand, too much alkaline can create an excess of bicarbonate that may also lead to other medical complications ("Biocarbonate Complications" Emedicine.MedScape.com).

According to AlkalizeForHealth.net most children's blood test at pH 7.5 (alkaline), half of adults are pH 6.5 or lower, and cancer patients are usually 4.5 (very acidic) or lower. This very acidic measurement presents another controversy: Cancer always seems to flourish in a body with excessive acid.

The fact that children have a natural basic alkaline state does support the science of alkaline being best for our bodies.

A natural pH balance in the bloodstream is activated with a buffer against acid. The calcium phosphate in our bones is part of that buffering system, which is another reason why an acidic state is a contributing factor in osteoporosis (AlkalizeForHealth.net).

This buffer is created by a homeostatic mechanism that is supposed to keep the blood pH at 7.4. It creates the depositing and withdrawing of acid and alkaline minerals from areas of the body like bones, soft tissue, body fluids and saliva, to maintain proper blood pH.

The conflicting research and interpretations surrounding different pH requirements is confusing for most of us. Add to that the misinformation campaigns between competitors, and it becomes intensified confusion for many. All of this scientific and opinionated misunderstanding continues to fuel the flames of this controversy.

alkalosis

Generally, alkalosis can occur when the pH of the blood exceeds 7.45. One of the most common causes is anxiety. Respiratory alkalosis is usually caused by hyperventilation, while Metabolic alkalosis may result from too much vomiting, causing a loss of hydrochloric acid (Merck Manual). Severe dehydration can also cause this condition.

According to Deborah Page Johnson in her book "Home Test pH Kit" the bottom line is that both acidosis and even alkalosis takes form as a result of an over-acid condition. LabTestsOnLine. org agrees, listing both conditions as an acid-based disorder.

Some of the following alkaline symptoms are: Nausea, vomiting, confusion, stupor or coma, hand tremor, muscle twitching or spasms and cramps, light-headedness, numbness or tingling in the face or extremities (Health.Google.com/health/ref/Alkalosis). If any of these things occur, use the urine "dipstick tests" with litmus paper, for a pH reading to see if your body is over-alkalized.

There are 53 recognized medical conditions that may be caused by alkalosis. There are also 14 medications, which can cause this condition. Additionally, there are 107 drugs listed which when combined with too much calcium creates alkalosis (http://www.wrongdiagnosis.com/symptoms/alkalosis/causes.htm). So ask your doctor if any medications you are taking contributes to this problem.

Understanding the delicate pH balance needed by the body is the key here before overindulging on anything including healthy alternatives. Our bodies need to be slightly alkaline, not over-alkaline.

water intoxication

News reports have shown stories about people who have died of apparent water overdose. That type of news may keep some people from drinking enough water, as most people don't know any more than the newscasters who are reading off the tele-prompter.

I have heard of this water-killing excuse from dehydrated persons who drink little water because of the fear of dying. The fact is water overdose deaths are very rare. The average person should not worry about such things unless they enter a water-drinking marathon.

Water intoxication is known as "hyper-hydration." Listed as a fatal disturbance in brain functions caused by an electrolyte imbalance produced by drinking too much water. This in turn can create kidney failure and death.

Kidney disorders also can strongely affect electrolyte balance. Additionally, drinking too much water can flush an abundance of toxins into the kidneys all at once, intensifying a kidney problem. There are also other disorders, some rare, that affect electrolyte balance. None are a medical mystery.

The point here is that a water overdose may be dangerous to a few persons depending on the health condition and water deficiencies of those individuals.

According to the MayoClinic.com, we all need at least eight 8-ounce glasses of water per day. To be more precise, body weight divided in half equals ounces needed. This is referred to as the 8x8 rule. If a person weighs 100 pounds they would only require 50 ounces of water. Divide that by eight-ounces, equals 48 ounces or about six 8-ounce glasses. A 180 pound person would require 90 ounces of water divided by eight-ounces, equals 11 eight-ounce glasses.

Keep in mind when dehydration is a way of life for many years, a safety precaution should be seriously observed. A parched person should slowly re-hydrate so the kidneys will safely adjust to avoid damage. Go easy at first!

testing water purity levels

Current research proves that most of our water supply is not pure. There are reports listing seven thousand industrial and agriculture chemicals that are known to infect our water. As well, the EPA is aware of the possible thousands of contaminates not currently regulated but known to be in some tap water.

Also according to the EPA, it is impossible to test for the additional 119 chemicals for which health-based limits have been set and impractical for me, so I settled for the simple pH test.

To test your tap water for more than pH, the most useful and common instrument is the Total Dissolved Solids (TDS) device that is designed to measure the amount of substances dissolved in water. They can easily be found on the Internet.

After testing numerous bottled waters and filtered tap water with the pH Test Liquid, I found many leaned toward alkaline. This often indicates the presence of inorganic minerals. However, tap water being what it is, may always have numerous contaminates regardless of any present filtering system.

The most recent study from The Environmental Working Group, which involved the analysis of 20 million water quality tests over a five-year period, shows that many local and regional water sources have up to 316 toxic chemicals.

Yet, regardless of the ever-present water pollutants, Dr. Batmanghelidj felt that drinking any water is better than no water at all. I agree with this point because the chemicals in our water would take longer to affect us than having no water in our bodies. Our odds for a longer life are better by drinking almost any kind of water.

water wise

So, what's all the fuss about? There are expensive and over-priced machines which will separate acid from alkaline, filters which clean up some of the toxins, oxygenated, ozonated, reverse osmosis and distilled, all of which are now common in the water market place.

What are you hoping for when choosing water to drink? Years of research motivated me to uncover a low cost alkaline formula using the purity of distilled water that I trust. Since the purifying process changes the water to an acidic base, I add a pinch of one mineral that converts the acid to alkaline.

The formula? I take two and a half gallons of distilled water and add at least an eighth teaspoon of Coral Calcium. Shake it up and let the molecules fully blend together. Other alkaline minerals are magnesium; potassium and sodium but healthy Coral Calcium is pre-digested for easy absorption, which builds bone density.

This formula gives me the purity of distilled alkaline water plus one of the most important elements for the bones, absorbable calcium. If you use coral calcium supplements for this, read the label as they are usually mixed with fillers or have chemical elements added which usually implies a low grade of coral. A trusted source for pure food grade Coral Calcium is from the original importers at CoralCalcium.com. They have it without fillers. It has noticeably strengthened my bones and fingernails.

Other alkalizing agents such as lemons, limes, apple cider vinegar, cayenne and/or arrowroot will also work. If Coral Calcium does not fit a budget, organic Arrowroot is my choice. It's nutritious and cost effective at MountainRoseHerbs.com.

Arrowroot is an herb once widely used in baby formulas. With a superior carbohydrate, it is the only starch with a Calcium Ash, perfect for a balanced body pH. Also it's high in Vitamin B6, Folate, Thiamin, Iron, Phosphorus, Niacin, Potassium and Manganese.

Arrowroot has also been known to alleviate diarrhea, nausea and vomiting. It's easy on the stomach with the ability to improve hydration by using it's moisture absorbing properties. I assume this increases hydration simply by holding water longer in our body, unlike a diuretic.

When you learn to read labels with vague verbiage in a clever arrangement of words geared to gain your trust, you will be able to spot the deceptive words on processed items even from health food markets.

Both sides of issues may have the same verbal skills to convince shoppers that their products are from honest humanitarian marketers with proprietary formulas, which are good for the world. The word "proprietary" also indicates that the manufacturers are not obligated to reveal the total ingredients in their packaged products.

One thing I have learned about health is not to believe the spoken or written word of anyone, even if the hearsay is backed-up with pieces of research. Conduct your own research, decide for yourself and see if it works for you. Be well. Drink hearty.

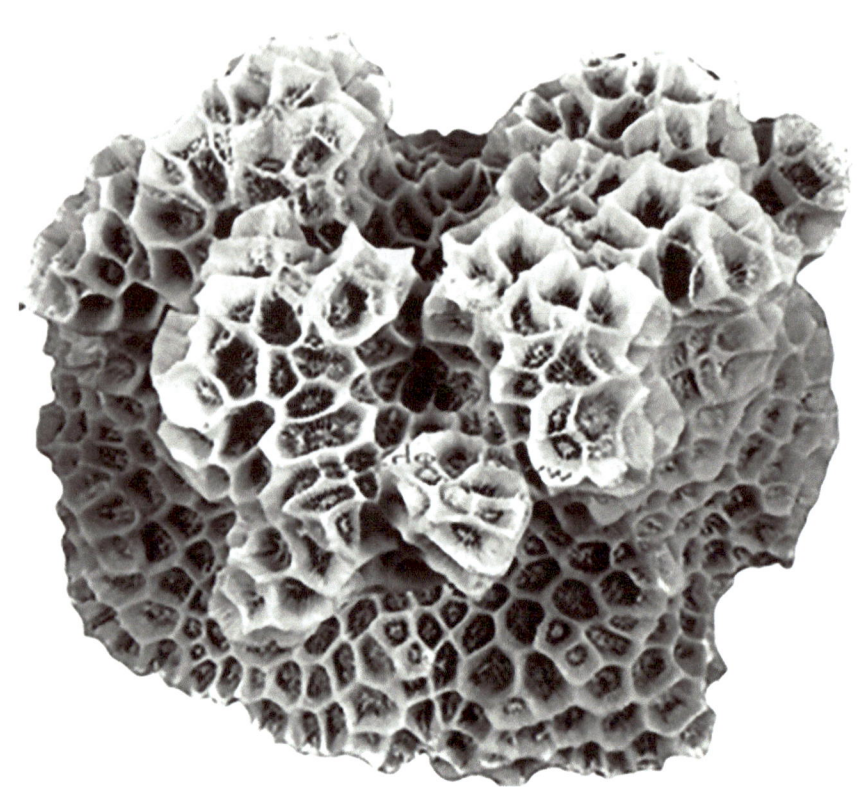

**coral calcium
up close**

alkaline water formula

Create Your Own Alkaline Water at Home

A. Two and a half gallons of distilled water
B. Add at least an eighth teaspoon of Coral Calcium
   or Arrowroot
C. Shake it up and let the molecules fully blend together

Other alkaline minerals are magnesium; potassium and
sodium but Coral Calcium is pre-digested for easy
absorption, which builds bone density.

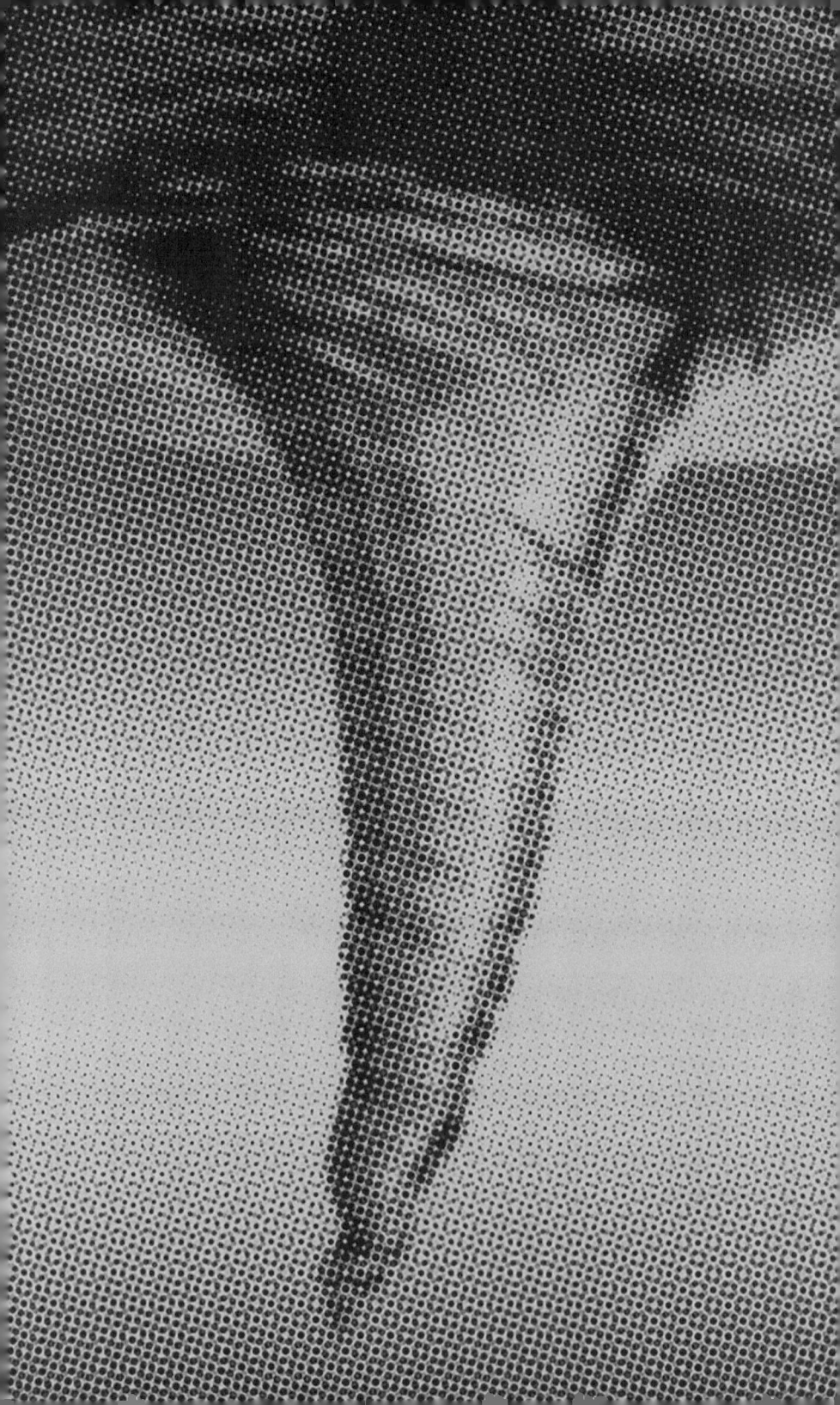

living water

Here I would like to mention two famous researchers. Vicktor Schauberger, who introduced the "living water" principle many years ago and Masuru Emoto whose research has indicated that water may be a living organism.

schauberger's water vortex

By creating a vortex spin at the bottom of a polluted pond, Schauberger showed it cleared up the water. This method drew in more oxygen but also reportedly created micro-clustering of the water. How important is that?

Our cells have clustered water in them at birth. Micro-clustering is structured water found in springs and in our bodies. Water is unique due to the way the H_2O molecules interact with each other. The special properties of water stem from the tendency of these molecules to associate, which form long and short-term clusters that undergo continued rearrangements.

How can water form these associations without being a living organism? More controversy.

The self-cleaning spirals and vortexes of a natural mountain stream create "Living waters." Rapidly moving streams also contain high levels of oxygen. Researchers suggest that a "spin" cools, softens, cleanses, oxygenates, polishes and re-energizes water. Plus, the chlorine evaporates more rapidly than water (Sulis-Health.co.uk).

Micro-clustering has become such a buzzword now, with glorified blenders being sold at high prices to spin drinking water. Just throw it in a blender for several minutes, that's vortex enough for me.

micro-clustering

There are more than a trillion molecules in a drop of water. Water in liquid form has various shapes in which hydrogen bonds are constantly being formed and broken into ever changing groupings referred to as clusters (PhysicalGeograhy.net). The molecular structure of water can be six-sided or hexagonal when it is frozen but not in liquid form according to various scientific sources.

The American Technologies Group claims to have discovered a unique type of stable, non-melting ice crystal "clusters." Adding any natural substance to agitating distilled water purportedly creates these ice crystals. Research has also shown that no matter how much water is used, it retains the biological activity of the substance added. This Homeopathy approach was deemed to be beyond the bounds of accepted science, yet Nobel Scientist Luc Montagnier, a virologist, recently discovered that water has a memory that continues even after many dilutions (NaturalNews.com).

Schauberger was the first to report that when water is forced through pipes or not exposed to a great deal of agitated movement, it becomes "dead." Then, when water is treated with a vortex spin it reportedly creates clustered molecules and brings the water back to life. This is another controversial issue. Yet, spinning does replicate the agitated movements of a natural water flow.

So, what if clusters are bigger, smaller, groups of six or scattered into ever-changing clusters? "Dead" tap water does have the large scattered clusters, which obviously should not absorb as well as micro-sized clusters. Whatever the case, dead or alive, drink water. Some of it is bound to get through.

As we grow older, because our bodies do lose the ability to absorb all the water we drink, our internal water levels decrease. Advocates believe that spinning water in a blender helps to create micro-clusters for easier penetration into our cells. The only suggestion I have is to drink it immediately while it is freshly energized.

The micro-clustering water sold in stores is reportedly electrically made, but normal water clustering depends on the motion of the water. There are now inexpensive systems available that will spin your water into your home.

masuru emoto

While Schauberger's living water principle was generally ignored for years, along comes Emoto to support this emerging research. Emoto photographically shows that water is a living thing that responds to external influences such as words, music, movement and even thoughts.

His most revealing test seems a bit like sci-fi. Emoto found that water responds to kind words such as "love and gratitude." He would take two cups of water from the same source and speak these words to just one cup. Placing them both in a microwave, he "nuked" the water. He would then freeze the two samples and photograph them under a microscope. The one not spoken to appeared dead, dark and ugly with no crystallization. The one exposed to the spoken words, crystallized like healthy water. These experiments could not be duplicated by other researchers. However, "belief" may have a lot to do with the results.

That sounds odd, yet beliefs about the nature of knowledge and learning appear to stimulate nearly all aspects of a person's daily life (Education Psychology Review "Vol6 #4 1994 Epistemological"). Epistemological Reports suggest that absolute beliefs will likely affect reasoning, learning and decision-making, but are often ignored in educational research.

This suggests that "belief" may even affect the results of some double-blind studies. This adds another possible reason for some of the conflicting water research. Inflexible mindsets are not objective. This applies to everyone.

Positive spoken words have a vibration ("The Biology of Belief" by Dr. Bruce Lipton). These vibrations may influence water, and according to this line of thinking, water may reflect the consciousness of the people living on this planet.

I suggest until someone comes up with a way to take all toxins out of our drinking supply and clean up the Earth's water pollution, look into Masuru Emoto's research. If communicating with water can lower the pollution levels of lake water in Japan, I would look at that with hope that part of the solution is also within our "belief" system.

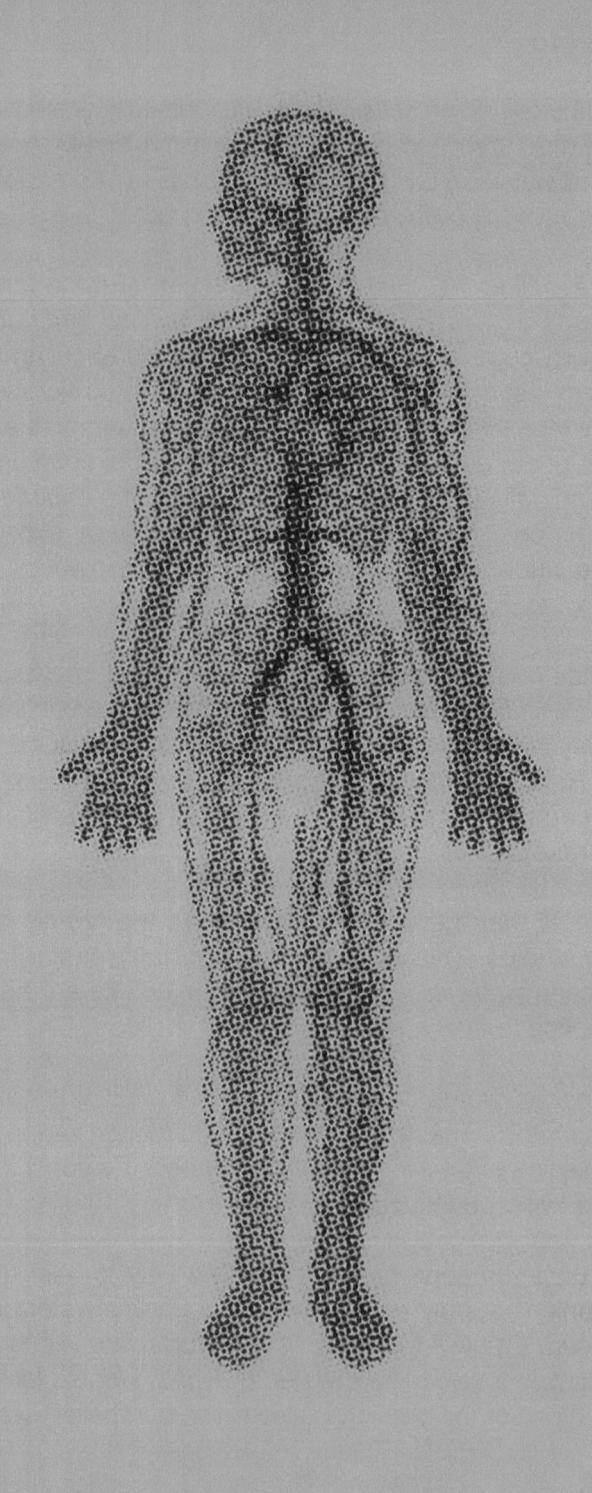

disease guide

Over the years while meeting with numerous individuals with health problems ranging from headaches, back and neck pain, stress, depression, high blood pressure, rheumatoid arthritis, colitis, dyspepsia and a host of other problems our bodies may develop in a lifetime, I found they all had one thing in common - dehydration.

Water is necessary for every function of the body. Without enough water, functions suffer and can even shut down. Adding to the list of problems that occur with dehydration are heart disease, leg pains, migraine, hangover pain, hypertension, and constipation.

water activates body mechanisms

With all the new developments and increased awareness in water conservation, we have rediscovered the importance of water. Like many people I was unaware of the body mechanisms that depend on water to avoid becoming dysfunctional.

Without water, the chemical reaction mechanism of hydrolysis suffers. Hydrolysis means water splitting. A vital process used for energy metabolism and storage, which all living cells need just to exist.

The brain is the control center for the body, and hydration is the fluid that makes it run efficiently. Energy generated by water is needed to manufacture "energy pools" for elemental exchanges for vital functions such as neuron-transmissions. Our consciousness depends upon keeping our energy pools filled with water.

Water also produces a Cell Adhesive Material to bond together cell structures. Amazing! Water is elastic, which cells use like "glue" (PhysicalGeograhy.net).

Without **hydrated** delivery lines which are attached to our nervous system to transport water, our brain cells will not easily move message transmissions to nerve endings for use. Cell to cell communication is an essential mechanism. Whether long term or short, memory depends upon adequate hydration for optimal function and is an integral part of this water process.

cell voltage

Cell membranes create a capacitor for storing electrons. Electrons develop from things such as raw food, alkaline water and sunshine, which help turn these membranes into small batteries. The power supply of cells measures -20 millivolts to -25 millivolts (TennantInstitute.com). Chronic disease is accompanied by a loss of voltage. Nutrition without voltage does not work. As well, voltage without nutrition also does not work. Water makes it all come together for smooth sailing.

acid & anti-acids

Many of us have too much acid in our system. People freely take antacids to help reverse this condition. Many antacid remedies have aluminum in them. Since listed as a poison, I would not personally take any aluminum-based products. When tissues and organs accumulate aluminum, the result is toxicity and dysfunction (Emedicine.MedScape.com "Aluminum").

Whenever there is a lot of aluminum in the soil of a region, the local people seem to suffer from Alzheimer. Researchers have also found traces of aluminum in the brains of Alzheimer victims. Though not recognized by the medical community in general, their own research ("Controversial Claims About the Causes of Alzheimer's Disease" - www.webmd.com/alzheimers/guide/controversial-claims-risk-factors) turns up high amounts of aluminum in some autopsy studies of patients with this disease. Additional studies also show that foods with large amounts of aluminum may lead to dementia.

In the 1950's, aluminum utensils were very popular. My Grandmother bought a set to overcook her food in lots of water, which was her generation's custom as a caution against food poisoning. But my Mother did some research and discovered that aluminum was listed as a toxic metal. So, instead, she bought "steel" advertised as "waterless cooking utensils." Using very little water, she did not overcook the food, and had no aluminum residue in the meals. I am convinced that this was a major contributor to why we grew up a nutritionally healthy family.

acid reflux

Acid Reflux can be a very painful experience especially when it wakes you up from a sound sleep. Millions of people suffer from this. It happens when food or liquid moves backwards from the stomach up into the esophagus. This creates chest pain. This pain can increase when your stomach is lying at the same level as your chest. Sitting up helps to momentarily stop the onslaught from your stomach.

I suffered from this until I began drinking water every time it occurred. It nearly always relieved the pain. Occasionally, whenever the pain persisted, I would swallow a mouthful of Apple Cider Vinegar, which eliminates the discomfort.

Vinegar is presumed to be an acid by most people. But when Apple Cider Vinegar is digested, undergoing oxidation, it changes to an alkaline ash. This can then dilute the stomach acid ("The Benefits of Apple Cider Vinegar" - GlobalHealingCenter.com), which seems to be why it stops acid reflux pain every time I take a teaspon full of vinegar with a chaser of water.

arthritis

Many people suffer from arthritis in this country. I once met a person whose hands were curled up like claws because his arthritis was so advanced. His friends had pointed out that he had lost a foot in height in ten years from this condition. This was hard to believe.

How can a person shrink that much? Simple. Our spines have 24 moveable bones stacked up one on top of the other. Between each is a disc. That disc normally holds 88% water, which when combined all together makes up 33% of the height of a spine. Besides shrinking the length of the spinal column, Chronic Dehydration apparently will make you shorter. I told him about the water connection, but this man was opposed to drinking water.

Most arthritis victims I have met have told me that they seldom drink water or that they don't drink enough. They may not have succumbed to the condition if they were sufficiently hydrated.

Some insist that they do drink "fluids", but it is not the same as water. When I tell people about arthritis and the water connection, some defend their condition with such claims as "it's in the cartilage." It is true that the cartilage does suffer, but the surface around the cartilage is comprised of a liquid that is facilitated by adequate water consumption. The movement of our joints creates a vacuum that sucks in water circulating through the joint. This liquid lubricates all the moving joints in your body.

If water creates the fluid that rides between joints, when our bodies dehydrate over a period of time and that fluid is missing, then bone begins to rub against bone. This creates severe pain. According to Dr. Batmanghelidj, this is the first step to rheumatism and arthritis, which is supported by his case histories. There may be other factors that contribute to the pain as joints worsen, but this Doctor's personal experiences have convinced me that dehydration is the doorway to arthritis.

34

brittle bones

Women in America suffer from low bone density that leads to osteoporosis. Not enough calcium in the bones creates this problem but water is needed to deliver this mineral.

Brittle bone sufferers should also know that drinking too much milk is another reason for this condition, according to the American Fitness Professionals & Associates. Here is how it works: Calcium rich dairy products are also full of proteins. But excess protein weakens our bones by creating an acid in the blood, which in turn pulls calcium out of the bones.

While evidence reveals that high amounts of this mineral may even play a role in creating prostate cancer, low amounts could also reduce the risk of cancer. They recommend calcium moderation ("High Calcium Intake Linked to Prostate Cancer" www.Cancer.org - American Cancer Society). Again, here is that "slightly alkaline"/ "slightly acid" rule which applies.

Either way, it is essential to know that bones are where new cell production is created. All sides agree on that, so there is no controversy.

breathing & bronchitis

I was visiting my old friend Millie who was eighty-two years young and coughing a lot. She had trouble breathing and had been taking a prescription drug for it, which had temporarily relieved her symptoms. She had been telling me that she was drinking enough water, but when I asked her to drink a glass of water, she barely could swallow even one gulp. She had been telling me this because she wanted to please me. That is when I began to realize that many of the people I speak to about water, exaggerate upon the amount they consume. Keep track of the amount, then you will know for sure.

Millie began to increase her daily consumption of water, becoming accustomed to the taste again and her breathing difficulty dramatically improved. Why? According to clinical research, water helps the air ducts in the lungs to facilitate breathing. Also, people who suffer from bronchitis are given antihistamines. Antihistamines do not heal the problem, only the symptoms. Dehydration creates an over-production of histamines in the lungs that block the bronchial tubes. Water stops the over-production of histamines.

cancer

A client I had known was using different alternatives to avoid the doctor's scalpel. Her cancer condition had been going on for years. After suggesting she look at the principles of how to simplify health, she began using various cancer killing herbal formulas to help purify her blood. She eventually graduated to more water, real salt, minerals and phyto-chemicals.

Meanwhile, she had opted to have the exterior tumor removed and a small amount of chemotherapy applied. I thought it was a good idea to remove the ugly uncomfortable growth on her bottom. But because of her new regimen none of her hair fell out and she did not experience nausea. Her doctor was surprised.

After a year on these alternatives, two doctors gave her a clean bill of health. No more cancer in her blood. She had embraced a positive state of mind and willingly changed her lifestyle. Then her immune system healed her as it was designed to do.

cholesterol

Many people worry about their cholesterol levels. Cholesterol and dehydration have a common link. When too much cholesterol gets in between the cells it hinders the water flow. This increases the dehydration which then increases the cholesterol stuck in your veins. This is a circle of circumstance that raises the chance of arterial plaque or clogged arteries.

colitis

In the lower part of the abdomen, colitis pain can occur, signaling that your body is dehydrated. The processing of food through the large intestine requires a necessary amount of water. If you are dehydrated, the food will not pass easily through the intestines. This is how colitis pain and constipation are apparently connected.

common cold

I have not suffered from the acidic condition of a common cold for decades. I still get them occasionally, but I eat strawberries, or occasionally take a spoonful of baking soda to bring my body's pH into balance. Strawberries taste better and Strawberry Leaf Tea will also work. Either way, my colds are always eliminated with alkaline.

constipation

Many people who experience constipation are not aware that this condition generally is caused by dehydration. Water facilitates digestion. I grew up believing that water dilutes the digestion process, but it is essential for digestion. Drink water with your meals to see how you feel.

depression & chronic fatigue syndrome

What causes depression? There can be many contributing factors that relate to depression, but bad diets and medications are two of the more common ones. Research also suggests that depression can be activated through dehydration because water determines the health of the brain. When our brains are dehydrating and processing medication at the same time, it can create even more stress.

We are electrical creatures. Without water, the electrolytes in the brain will not flash efficiently. Body Fluids between cells maintain Voltages across Cell Membranes that carry Electrical Impulses to other cells (Health.HowStuffWorks.com). When there is not enough water to do this it can intensify stress. Plus, the flashing of lights in darken cells begin to burn out. Hydrating those water lines will again help to light up those flashing cells powered through the water canals that are built into our nerve pathways.

In certain scientific circles it has been concluded that dehydration in a depressive state may lead to chronic fatigue syndrome (CFS). Dehydration creates and stagnates our internal cleansing system (FatigueAnswers.com/dehydration.html). Therefore, energy is stalled and we get tired. There may be other reasons for CFS but the lack of enough water is part of the equation.

exhaustion

In the process of moving to another state, a friend called me to say she had been driving for several days and her ankles had swollen. She was having a great deal of pain. Although she had been drinking a lot of water, she had been suffering from a fever and perspired a great deal. When she went to a local hospital, they found that she was dehydrated and exhausted. Her blood vessels had shrunk and, combined with the exhaustion, had slowed the blood circulation in her legs while in a driving position, which caused the swelling. After adequate rest and substantial amounts of water, her body recovered.

heart attacks

A woman called me to ask about a 41-year-old friend who had died of a massive heart attack. The victim was very conscious of health, worked out daily, had eaten the right foods, regularly took vitamin supplements, and drank about a quart of fresh carrot juice a day. I asked if her friend drank enough water. She had not. Dehydration shrinks the arteries that carry blood to the heart. Being aware of your heart and the importance of drinking enough water for it to pump properly may save your life.

heartburn - gastritis - ulcers

I repeatedly run into people who get heartburn. Gastritis is a symptom of dehydration and diet.

Most of us mix our foods with other foods so our bodies are digestively confused and may not release any digestive fluids. This is another reason for gastritis. Drinking water with your mixed meals helps facilitate the action in your stomach. Alkaline water is better as it stimulates the production of acid for digestion.

Ulcers are also linked to dehydration. Dr. Batmanghelidj eliminated thousand of cases of ulcers by adding water to his treatments. Your stomach lining is better off by drinking water.

hypertension & high blood pressure

I met a fellow once who had a big stomach and red face and suffered from a terrible case of hypertension and high blood pressure. Besides a bad diet, high blood pressure is intensified by chronic dehydration. He was a heavy drinker and did not exercise, which helps relieve hypertension. When the body does not have enough water, blood vessels are constricted. I suggested drinking more water and reading Dr. Batmanghelidj's book. He wanted to argue about it. He was rigid in his ways and died shortly thereafter.

Dr. Batmanghelidj, after many years of practice, pointed out that the way modern medicine treats high blood pressure and hypertension is inadequate. In his own words "to the point of scientific absurdity."

lower back & neck pain

Recently I was visiting a friend who mentioned how he suffers from lower back pain. He was only thirty years old. Noting that his lips were very dry, I mentioned dehydration. He admitted he hardly ever drinks water. I told him that one of the lower disks floats on water that holds up most of the upper body. Without water, the weight of our body becomes supported on a "dry" disk, which produces the pain.

Many years ago I was involved in a traffic accident and my neck and lower back were injured. To this day, I still have a bend in my neck while normal people have curves. Winter was literally a pain in the neck. I usually took remedies to increase my blood circulation to ease the pain. Now that I am well hydrated, the neck and lower back are no longer a painful problem.

Also, to reduce pain faster check out MSM, known as the sulfur molecule, which helps lower pain levels. By using an abundance of this molecule, a chemical listed as non-toxic, it reversed 20 years of chronic nighttime body pain for me in a week.

I have a friend who sleeps on two or three pillows at once and complains of neck aches. Sleeping like that can create neck pain. The proper position for your neck during sleep helps to create adequate fluid circulation within the disk spaces. Sleeping on just one pillow while in a hydrated state can contribute to a better night of sleep.

lymphatic system

The lymphatic system is a network of vessels running through our entire body and is an important aspect of being healthy. These water highways and byways perform the vital function of cleaning the fluid surrounding our cells by removing impurities and waste products.

Water is essential for the lymphatic system, which depends on a constant supply of fluids to function at peak performance.

migraines

The brain shrinks when dehydrated, which creates migraines. Drinking sodas or coffee creates more dehydration. Coffee and soda are both acidic diuretics that elevate the rate of urination. If I drink coffee in the morning, after becoming wide awake from it, I drink water to replace the fluids lost from coffee's diuretic effect.

I had a client who had constant migraines and took all kinds of nutrients and medications for them. Although he would not be considered an alcoholic, he did enjoy a drink at day's end. I informed him that alcohol initiates cell dehydration in the brain that can cause frequent headaches and hangovers. By drinking water after the affects of liquor were felt, he later experienced milder headaches. In addition to dehydration, be aware that some individuals may suffer migranes triggered by foods containing the amino acid Tyramine; a full list of such foods can be easily obtained on the Internet.

morning sickness

How many of you know that a woman's morning sickness is a sign of dehydration for both the mother and the fetus? Instead of water, the future mother will take a prescription that may relieve the nausea but the drug may also aggravate the fetus and create more dehydration. This may lead to giving birth to a baby with medical problems.

water weight

Water weight? Some people do not drink enough water because they fear the possibility of gaining more weight. And some take diuretics that dehydrate them more. When the body is dehydrated it will retain as much water as possible to ensure survival.

We generally are led to believe it is the water adding to the weight, but usually it is because **you do not drink enough water**. Drinking the proper amount of water reduces water weight. Strange but provable.

What confuses the body is when thirst and hunger happens at the same time, we usually consume food first because we think we are hungry. Drinking water first, tends to separate these two sensations. Overeating may satisfy the urge for water but it also contributes to dehydration and weight gain.

I know a woman who began drinking several quarts of water a day and within two weeks she lost ten pounds. I suspect some of it was water weight because her body did not need to hold the water inside, because it was no longer in a drought condition. Plus drinking more water makes a person feel less hungry.

unknown diseases

Have you ever been told by a doctor that you have an unknown disease? Some doctors do not take into consideration the dehydration connection. According to Dr. Batmanghelidj, doctors are not trained to understand the importance of water. Instead, they are educated to use chemicals and surgery that may be helpful in specific cases, but does not correct the fundamental reason for your body's malfunctions, which often involves dehydration.

spiritual healing

Once I had an acquaintance who was a spiritual healer. She claimed that she was once helped through the process of "hands-on" healing while speaking in tongues, which she now practices and has a lot of faith in.

Despite all of her faith though, she was still chronically dehydrated. She did not like drinking water, so I asked her why she had not "cast out" her condition? She had no answer.

I am not suggesting giving up prayer if that is part of your life, but how many amongst us have that kind of devine power? That's why water was created, and for most of us only water can cast out dehydration.

about the author

Timothy Nicely has been researching health for more than 30 years. A published author and writer for several national magazines, he was fortunate to have interviewed numerous mainstream doctors and review their innovative books.

All of these exceptional doctors followed the Hippocratic oath by publishing their data for the enlightenment of society. Ultimately for the author, this knowledge helped to create the realization that staying healthy is simpler than assumed.

The author's humanitarian efforts as a mentor to children has earned him awards from the March of Dimes and the YMCA, as well as several Commendations from the City of Los Angeles.

references

Like a newspaper story, references are within the text to make it easier to search the sources of information.

All information used in this investigative approach adheres to the fair use rule regarding criticism, comments, news reporting, teaching, scholarship and research.

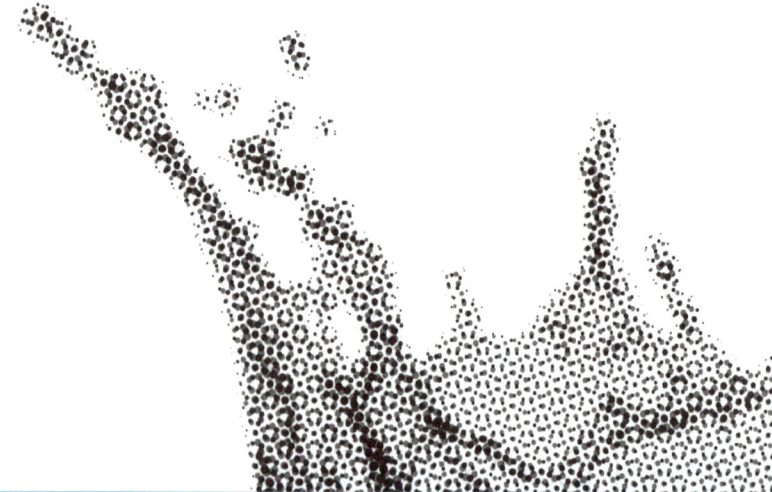

QUESTIONS / COMMENTS / SUGGESTIONS
Publisher@SimplifyYourHealth.org

www.ingramcontent.com/pod-product-compliance
Lightning Source LLC
Chambersburg PA
CBHW050843290526
45792CB00002B/504